Fonga Noutchia Placide Nelson

Emulsifying properties of shea butterProduced in Mali

Fonga Noutchia Placide Nelson

Emulsifying properties of shea butterProduced in Mali

ScienciaScripts

Cover image: www.ingimage.com

This book is a translation from the original published under ISBN 978-613-8-40645-7.

Publisher:
Sciencia Scripts
is a trademark of
Dodo Books Indian Ocean Ltd. and OmniScriptum S.R.L publishing group

120 High Road, East Finchley, London, N2 9ED, United Kingdom
Str. Armeneasca 28/1, office 1, Chisinau MD-2012, Republic of Moldova, Europe
Managing Directors: Ieva Konstantinova, Victoria Ursu
info@omniscriptum.com

Printed at: see last page
ISBN: 978-620-8-39913-9

DEDICATIONS AND THANKS

I dedicate this thesis ...
To the Eternal God Almighty,
I thank you Lord for your love, your works and your manifest presence in my life.
You were my support.

To my mother Mrs DJEUTCHA Colette,
In my life, for as long as I can remember, you have always been both mother and father. The man I am, the man I'm becoming, is largely the fruit of the inestimable sacrifices you made for us. Thank you for life, Mum, thank you for my life.
I hope you're a little prouder of me every day and that the good Lord allows us to live long enough. I work in the hope of seeing you happy and free of this worried and anxious era that you've always had. Find in this work mother
an expression of my eternal love.

To my late father, Mr Marc NOUTCHIA,

The ups and downs of life never allowed us to have and develop the bond that a father has and can develop with his son. I hope that you have found peace from where you are and that you are watching over us. I hope that my daily choices follow an ideal that you might have had. May your soul rest in peace, Dad.

To my big sister, the late NDAMDJEU Corine Virginia,

Departed at a very young age and in troubled circumstances, may your soul rest in peace.

To Papa Adolphe Watat,
Dad, you were always able to pass on to us the rigour of a job well done, the determination and patience to achieve our goals. Your wise and noble fatherly advice has guided and enlightened my daily steps and choices. This work is also yours. Thank you for believing and for allowing me to reach the end of this achievement.

To dad, Jean-Marie TCHIENKOUA,
You have been like my biological father because of your unfailing support at difficult and perplexing times throughout my life. Please find in this work the expression of my warmest feelings and deepest love.

To Cyriaque YANOU and Ivane DJAMEN,
As a token of my brotherly affection, my deep tenderness and gratitude, I wish you a life full of happiness, success and health.

May Almighty God protect you and keep you.

To all my aunts and uncles,

As a token of my attachment and high regard. I hope that you will find in this work the expression of my warmest feelings.

May this work bring you the esteem and respect that I hold for you, and be proof of your commitment to the cause.
of the desire I have always had to honour you. Best wishes for health and happiness.

To my dear cousins,
Please find in this work the expression of my deepest respect and affection most sincere.

To Dr Nadia ZOUNA,

More than a big sister, you have been Nadia, a friend, an advisor and finally a mother. My first steps in Bamako were guided by you. Thank you for the welcome and for the way you showed me, for the sympathy and affection you always showed me. Woman a fighter, you remained a source of inspiration for me.

My family from Bamako,

Dr Nadia, Dr Andrea, Dr Maurine, Dr Ida, Dr Diane, Aude, Carole, Chorine, Trésor, Adam, Tatiane, Christian. Thank you for the pleasant moments we spent together. May God grant you happiness, health and success.

My elders,

Dr Berthol TIODO, Dr Éric ESSO, Dr Flaure LATAGUIA, Dr Estelle KAMGA, Dr Tatiana, Dr MONKAM Goliath, Dr Kevin NIASSAN, Dr John WAANI, Dr Adrien FOGANG, OMBAHO Francis

Thank you for your help and advice. Your consideration for me and your generosity will bear fruit.

My cadets,

Chorine, Romeo, Ingrid, Naomie, Cyrielle, Jaurès, Christian, Valérie, Michelle, Dimitri, Benjamin, Manuela, Lucrèce, Fortune, Lunelle, Flora

Thank you for your warmth, friendship and support.

My comrades,

Joel DJEKEU, Dr Faouziya ADAMA, Dr Ines LOWE, Aimé SIEWE, Yétina, junior, Tatiana

Thank you for the time spent together. Many thanks to Dr Ida Ngongang,
My cousin, who over the years has become more than a sister, thank you for your presence and support over all these years. May the Most High lead us and enable us to achieve more than our goals.

To the HDB Hospital Pharmacy Dr MARIKO, Nouh, Sibri, Mai, My sister,
Thank you for enriching my knowledge and for the trust you have placed in me.
May God grant you long life.

To the MARSEILE promotion,

It has been a pleasure for me to share these years together. May the good Lord guide us as we go forward.

To the thirteenth class of the FAPH/ Bamako numérus clausus,

It has been a pleasure for me to share these years together. May the good Lord guide us for the future.

AT AEESCM,

Thank you for your welcome, solidarity and integration.

To Josiane MAWABO,

As the years go by, the enigma remains almost intact "Laughs". I wish you a life full of happiness, success and health.

To the PETON family,

In memory of the times we spent together, please find in this work the expression of my deepest respect and my most sincere affection. Thank you for your hospitality and generosity over the years.

To my supervisors,

Thank you for your teaching and guidance over the years.

To my co-director Dr. Aichata Ben Adam MARIKO,

This work is first and foremost yours. It has been an honour to work with you. Your rigour in the scientific approach, your availability, your support at all times and at any moment, and your sense of understanding have all been very useful in bringing this work to a successful conclusion. Thank you, dear Master.

To all the people who took part in the preparation of this work To all those whom I have

failed to mention

TRIBUTES TO THE MEMBERS OF THE JURY

To our Master and Chairman of the jury Professor Elimane MARIKO

➯ Honorary Professor of Pharmacology at the Faculty of Pharmacy and the Faculty of Medicine and Odontostomatology (FAPH /FMOS);

➯ The Malian army's first pharmacist;

➯ Former Colonel Major of the armed forces, defence and veterans ;

➯ President of the Association des Ressortissants de la Commune Rurale de Tomba ;

➯ Former head of the HIV-AIDS coordination unit at the Ministry of Defence and Veterans Affairs;

➯ Former United Nations official in the fight against HIV/AIDS in the Democratic Republic of Congo;

➯ Rector of the Free Scientific University of Bamako (USLB);

➯ Officer of the National Order of Mali. Dear Master,

You are doing us a great honour by agreeing to chair this jury, despite your busy schedule.

Your simplicity and humility are qualities that make you a master envied by all. Please accept the expression of our deep gratitude and respect.

May Allah the good Lord grant you long life and good health.

To our Master and Judge

Doctor Hamma Boubacar MAÏGA

➯ Assistant Master in Galenic Pharmacy ;

➯ Head of the FAPH clinical training monitoring committee

;

➯ Pharmacist at Mali Hospital;

➯ Member of the scientific committee of the Mali Hospital.

Dear Master,

You have done us an immense honour by agreeing to judge this work.

We were deeply impressed by your approachability, your generosity, your availability and your sense of a job well done.

Please accept our sincere gratitude

To our Master and Judge

Dr Bakary M CISSE

➯ Senior Assistant in Galenic Pharmacy ;

➯ Lecturer and researcher at the National Health Laboratory;

➯ Secretary for the organisation of the Collectif des Pharmaciens Enseignants Chercheurs ;

➯ Member of the Société Ouest Africaine de Pharmacie Galénique et Industrielle.

Dear Master,

We would like to thank you for the simplicity with which you agreed to sit on our thesis jury.

We were touched by the kindness with which you received us. By agreeing to judge this work, you have done us a great honour. Please accept the expression of our most distinguished consideration.

To our Master and thesis co-director

Dr. Aichata MARIKO

➯ Doctor of Pharmacy ;

➯ Research assistant/teacher at the Faculty of Pharmacy (FAPH) ;

➯ Galenic Pharmacist, Head of the Hospital Pharmacy Department at

Bamako Dermatology Hospital;

➯ Master's degree in biomedical sciences with a focus on dermopharmacy and cosmetology from the Université Libre de Bruxelles;

➯ Master's degree in drug science and health with a major in Biopharmacy, Pharmaceutical Engineering and Formulation from the University of Ouaga I Pr KI-ZERBO.

Dear Master,

Your rigour in your work, your love of a job well done and your strong sense of duty have won our admiration. This work is the fruit of your desire to improve, your availability and above all your know-how. Your punctuality, self-confidence, humility and sociability make you a woman of exceptional class, always ready to listen to and care for others. Thank you for your patience, your encouragement, your support at all times and, above all, your sound advice, which helped to fuel our thinking. You will remain for us an example to follow.

Words fail us when it comes to thanking you for all you have done for our training to make us good pharmacists.

Please accept our deepest gratitude.

To our Master and Thesis Director

Professor Ousmane FAYE

➮ ***Master of lectures agrégé à the Faculty of Medicine and of Odontostomatology ;***

➮ ***Specialist in Dermato-Lepro-Venereology ;***

➮ ***PhD in Public Health and Biomedical Information Science from***

Pierre and Marie Curie University;

➮ ***Former Vice Dean of the FMOS ;***

➮ ***Co-ordinator of the TELEDERMALI project.***

Dear Master,

It's a great honour and a real pleasure for us to have you as one of our partners.

director of this work, despite your many commitments.

The welcome you gave us did not leave us indifferent.

Your kindness, your human warmth, your enthusiasm and your scientific rigour make you a man of undeniable qualities.

Please accept our sincere gratitude.

May the Most High give you health and long life.

TABLE OF CONTENTS

INTRODUCTION

The Shea tree or "Shea yiri", meaning "tree of life" in the Bambara vernacular, is a plant native to the arid regions of sub-Saharan Africa [1]. Unrefined shea butter is the oleaginous substance obtained from the kernel of the nuts of Vitellaria paradoxa C.F. Gaertn, a member of the Sapotaceae family, using manual or mechanical methods [2]. Known for thousands of years, this butter is a highly prized resource among African populations, who already used it as a plant medicine for its anti-inflammatory, anti-haemorrhoidal, relaxing, cough-relieving, antioxidant and healing properties, etc. In addition to these medical properties, shea butter also has other properties, which is why it is used in cosmetics, particularly in body care for its emollient, moisturising, hair care, baby and mother care, photo-protective properties and to prevent stretch marks... Butter was also used as food and as a raw material in the manufacture of soaps for domestic use (kabacorouni in the Bambara vernacular). Today, this fat is highly prized by both the cosmetics and pharmaceutical industries because of its special composition, which gives it the physical and chemical properties (melting point, easy spreading) and therapeutic properties already mentioned [3-7]. It represents a source of monetary wealth for the African populations living in the shea belt, particularly in rural areas. Nigeria, Burkina Faso and Mali remain the world's leading exporters of this product [8]. Several studies have been carried out on the physico-chemical properties of shea butter, but very little data exists on its emulsifying properties. One study entitled "Détermination expérimentale de la valeur de la balance hydrophile / lipophile requise du beurre de karité" carried out at the Laboratoire du développement du médicament (LADME) at the Université Pr Ki Zerbo in Ouagadougou, suggested that shea butter might have emulsifying properties and recommended that further research be carried out in this area [9]. To initiate this research, a number of questions need to be raised: How does shea butter act as a stabiliser? What would be the optimum quantities for stabilising emulsions? How long will the emulsions remain stable? We plan to conduct a study on the possible emulsifying properties of shea butter. The aim of this work is to highlight the possible emulsifying properties of shea butter with a view to its use as an emulsifier or co-emulsifier. If confirmed, this hypothesis could provide a wealth of information for manufacturers and consumers. This would allow :

➢ Reduce the cost of manufacturing emulsions, as butter is an economically accessible resource

➢ To be used as a co-emulsifier in the manufacture of W/O emulsions in order to increase the stability of emulsions containing it and reduce the quantity of surfactants to be used.

➢ To make the most of Africa's natural resources and to be in the the green cosmetics movement

➢ To reinforce the studies already carried out on the physical and chemical properties of shea butter.

OBJECTIVES

General objective :

Study the emulsifying properties of shea butter in Mali.

Specific objectives

1- Formulating water/shea butter emulsions ;

2- Quantify the shea butter needed to stabilise emulsions;

3- Estimate the minimum time required to guarantee emulsion stability.

GENERAL

1. General information on shea butter

1.1. History of shea

Shea is a traditionally and exclusively African product. The first written records of this product were brought back by the Scottish explorer Mungo Park in 1796 in the region of Ségou (Mali), who was the first to give the botanical characteristics of this tree, as well as listing the main applications of shea butter in his 1797 work entitled "Travels in the Interior Districts of Africa". In this document, Park describes a product transported to the coast of Gambia: "shea- toulou", which literally means "tree butter" or "vegetable butter". He explains that in all places, the local population is involved in gathering the fruit and preparing the butter, which is obtained by cooking the almonds in boiling water. This traditional method of production is still used today.

In 1999, researchers at the POS pilot plant - a private research facility in Saskatoon - and their colleagues in Burkina Faso began examining ways to improve the processing and cleaning of shea. The research was undertaken as part of a $1.5 million initiative funded by Canada to improve the shea butter and kernel trade in the West African country of Burkina Faso. According to Pierre Zaya [11], a shea specialist at the International Development Research Centre (IDRC) in Ottawa, "there is no shea industry as such in Burkina Faso".
". Researchers in Saskatoon and Ouagadougou, the capital of Burkina Faso, have decided to get things moving and help the country develop its own shea industry. In 1987, two studies were carried out on the chemistry of shea kernels and butter by Zénabou CISSÉ [12] and the evolution of the physico-chemical parameters of shea butter by Alfred TRAORÉ and Adama BARRO [13] in Burkina Faso. Their contributions have led to a better understanding of the properties of shea butter and its behaviour as a function of treatment and storage, the influence of pulping, temperature, drying method, extraction method and the state of the kernels on the butter and acidity content. From 1988 to 1998, the Institut de l'environnement et de recherches agricoles [14], with the help of its team of mechanical engineers and chemists and with the participation of women shea producers, developed equipment adapted to the extraction of shea butter (mill, crusher, roaster, press, washing system and shea use filter).

The most recent statistical data on shea is provided by the Food and Agriculture Organization of the United Nations [15]. The information is available for 7 of the 16 shea-producing countries and goes up to 2003. The topics covered are: description of the tree, the fruit, the composition of the butter, the origin and history of shea, growing conditions, yields, the main causes of crop destruction, quality criteria at world level and minimum requirements for importing the kernels, sectors of use: the chocolate industry, cosmetology and pharmacology, markets, the shea industry, technology: traditional methods, pressing and solvent extraction, price trends for shea kernels and butter, e-commerce and economic policies. Research on the influence of almond processing methods on shea butter quality was carried out by a group of researchers in Cameroon, and the scientific article was published on the PBA: Procédés Biologiques et Alimentaires website on 30 May 2005 [16]. This is the study most closely related to this master's project.

1.2. Description of shea butter

1.2.1. Definition

Shea butter is a vegetable oil, an edible substance extracted from the fruit of the shea tree, which grows mainly in the wooded savannahs of West, Central and East Africa, and whose name means "life" in the Mandinka language [17]. Shea butter is mainly consumed in traditional cooking or used in the chocolate industry in Europe as a substitute for cocoa butter. It is best known in Africa, Europe and the United States for its skin-softening and nourishing cosmetic properties. As a result of these properties, it is now used in many cosmetic and pharmaceutical products.

1.2.2. Shea tree

The plant species Vitellaria paradoxa C. F. Gaertn, whose synonym is Butyrospermum parkii (G. Don) or Butyrospermum paradoxa subsp.parkii (G. Don) Hepper, is known as "karité" in French and "shea" in English. It is a Sudano-Sahelian agroforestry species in the order Ebenales and family Sapotaceae [5].

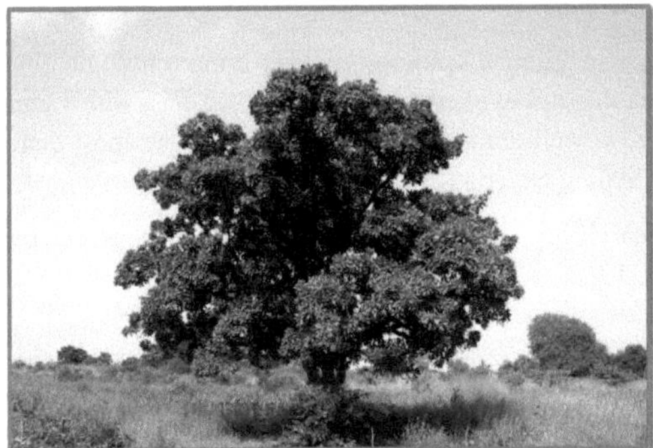

Figure 1: Shea tree

The shea tree is around 15 metres tall, with a thick trunk up to 150 centimetres (cm) in diameter, stocky branches (with thick bark) and dense, deciduous foliage (Figure 3). The leaves, grouped in large, tight clumps, pubescent and rusty red in their youth, gradually become hairless, leathery, shiny and dark green. Flowering, characterised by groups of 30 to 40 highly fragrant yellowish flowers, generally takes place from April to May. The fruit is a yellow-green or yellow elliptical berry, 3 to 6 cm long and weighing on average 20 to 25 grams (g). It contains one, two or three seeds called "shea nuts" [18,19]. The tree is found mainly in Africa, in wooded savannah, stretching from the Senegal-Sudan border to Central Africa, through southern Mali, Burkina Faso, northern Togo, Ghana, Benin, Côte d'Ivoire, Nigeria, southern Chad and Sudan. It inhabits the savannahs and dry forests from Guinea to Sudan, a strip 5,000 km long and 400 km wide. 750 km wide, covering an area of 1 million km², this zone is nicknamed the "shea belt" by traders.

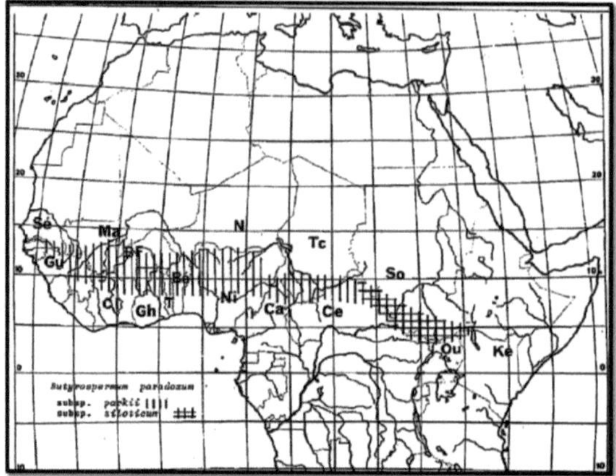

Figure 2: Distribution of shea in Africa [21].

It grows spontaneously in arid and semi-arid regions, with rainfall ranging from 500 to 1,500 millimetres (mm) and climates marked by two distinct seasons, with a long dry period. It also grows spontaneously on well-drained lateritic soils [18]. The most densely populated shea soils are found from Mali to Nigeria [21,22].

Recent scientific research has also shown that shea cultivation in our regions is technically possible and feasible [19].

1.2.3. Manufacture

Sixteen million African women in rural areas are responsible for harvesting the fruit, extracting it and marketing it locally [23,24], hence its nickname "women's gold". However, the international shea industry is essentially dominated by men [24-26]. "Shea butter is an essential ingredient in the diet and informal trade in the areas where it is produced" [24].Traditionally, the pulp is removed from the shea fruit, which is harvested between mid-June and mid-September. This produces a nut from which the kernel is recovered. It is washed and left to dry, then crushed, roasted, ground and churned. Three kilos of almonds yield about one kilo of butter, a ratio of one third [27]. There are three methods for extracting the butter from the shea kernel:

a) The traditional method

The almonds are crushed, roasted and ground to a thick paste, which is then vigorously churned in water. Immersion in boiling water separates the butter from the other components of the almond, in particular the impurities that settle to the bottom of the container. Once removed, the butter floating on the surface is kneaded before being cooked for a long time to allow the water to evaporate and the impurities to settle. The oil (in fact the liquid butter) thus obtained is filtered before being packaged. This produces artisanal shea butter, but the heat somewhat alters its qualities.

The result is 30 to 35% butter per dry weight of nuts [27].

b) Extraction by cold pressing

The kernels are simply crushed in a press at a temperature below 80°C. This mechanical method does not extract all the butter from the nut, but it is the method that gives the best quality, since the active ingredients of the shea butter are preserved.

c) Solvent extraction

The almonds are ground and then a solvent, hexane, is used. The butter still contained in the almonds dissolves in the hexane. The hexane is then allowed to evaporate and the shea butter is recovered. This method is the most profitable, but the shea butter obtained is of inferior quality. The result is up to 45% butter per dry weight of nut [27].

d) In the West

Most butter and butter components are imported in the form of processed kernels from the West and Asia, which deprives producing countries and traditional processors of a significant proportion of the added value in the industry [28]. "Shea butter is extracted using industrial processes, mainly in Europe, and then separated into two fractions:

- A vegetable fat fraction (stearin): sold for the formulation of cocoa butter equivalents or improvers (CBE/CBI) and margarines.
- And a fraction of oil, used as a cheap base in the production of margarines, as well as a component of animal feed" [27].

This olein is also sold to cosmetics manufacturers, and despite intensive marketing campaigns on the beneficial effect of the sector on women's empowerment, it accounts for 50% of the shea used in the cosmetics industry [28].

1.2.4. Composition

Shea butter contains five main fatty acids (triacylglycerides): palmitic, stearic, oleic, linoleic and arachidic acids. Of these, stearic and oleic acids account for around 85-90%, depending on origin [29,30]:

- Oleic acid (40-60%)
- Stearic acid (20-50%)
- Linolenic acid (3-11%)
- Palmitic acid (2-9%)
- Linoleic acid (< 1%)
- Arachidic acid (< 1%)

The relative proportions of stearic and oleic acids influence the consistency of butter [30]. Stearic acid gives a solid consistency, while oleic acid gives a soft or even liquid consistency. For example, shea butter from the Mossi plateau (Burkina Faso) and from northern Ghana has a higher stearic acid content and is therefore generally harder; shea butter from Uganda is liquid and requires fractionation to become butter; shea butters from West Africa are more variable in consistency [30]. In addition to its fatty acids, shea butter contains catechises, vitamins E and A, essential fatty acids [31] and triterpenes [32].

1.2.5. According to origin

The geographical origin of shea butter influences its composition [30]. In fact, several studies, including one by Ben Gurion University of the Negev, show "high variability between provenances from different African regions and a significant effect of climate on levels of α-tocopherol" (a form of vitamin E). "Total tocopherol content (α, β, γ and δ) in 102 shea butter samples from 11 countries ranged from 29 to 805 μg/g shea butter, with an average of 220 μg/g. α-Tocopherol, the main form detected, constitutes on average 64% of the total tocopherol content." Shea trees from "Vitellaria located in hot, dry climates have the highest levels of α-tocopherol (for example, an average of 414 ng/g in samples from N'Djamena, Chad). The lowest concentrations of α-tocopherol (are) found in samples from cold mountainous regions, particularly in the north of the country (an average of 29 μg/g)" [33]. The same applies to stearic acid and triterpene alcohol content (mainly amyrins, lupeol and butyrospermol), according to a Japanese study [34]. Oleic acid is dominant in shea butter from Uganda, while stearic acid is dominant in shea butter from West Africa, according to an Italian study of 150 regions in Mali, Burkina Faso, Nigeria and Uganda [35]. French results show "differences between East and West Africa in the fat composition of shea nuts: eastern nuts (have) a significantly higher fat and oleic acid content" based on samples from "624 trees in five African countries (Senegal, Mali, Burkina Faso, Ghana and Uganda)" [36].

1.2.6. Socio-economic importance of shea butter in Mali

a) Offer

According to Brèves de la Revue Marchés Tropicaux et Méditerranéens in 2008, shea supplies from Mali were distributed as follows in 2005:

Table I: Shea supply from Mali

Elements	Quantities in tonnes
Nuts	85000
Almond	8000
Butter	500

Mali is the world's second largest producer of shea nuts after Nigeria, and ranks sixth in terms of exports. According to the FAO, Mali produced 190,000 tonnes of shea nuts in 2008. This compares with an estimated potential of 250,000 tonnes for the same year, giving an overall production of shea nuts equal to 76% of the estimated potential. As far as exports are concerned, the latest available data on FAOSTAT estimates that 4,015 tonnes of walnuts were produced in 2002, compared with 2,432 tonnes in 2004 [37].

Table II: Shea butter production and exports

Year Mali	1998	2000	2002	2004	2006	2008
Production	85000	85000	85000	85000	70000	190000
Export			4015	2432		

According to the DNSI (Direction Nationale de la Statistique et de l'Informatique) 2003, 3.5% of Malian exports are shea nuts. It accounts for 81% of oilseed exports. Two-thirds of these exports go to the sub-regional market (Republic of Côte d'Ivoire, Burkina Faso and Ghana), which markets it under their own labels. European manufacturers using shea as a raw material are well represented in these countries. According to the national PCDA programme (Competitiveness and Agricultural Diversification Programme), the production potential of the Malian production base is estimated in the following table:

Table III: Potential supply in Mali (PCDA)

Estimation of shea stock	408,607,769 feet
Estimated surface area	229,912,500 ha
Potential production	250.000 t
Potential collection	150.000 t
Estimated consumption	97.000 t
Total estimated export	53.000 t
Export in the form of shea kernels	50.000 t
Export in the form of shea butter	3.000 t

b) The request

Demand for Malian shea butter is mainly local, national and sub-regional. There are no data available on the demand for shea butter at any level. The few data we have on national consumption are as follows old. They date back to 1993 with a study by APROMA which highlighted that, on average, a family of 7 consumes the equivalent of 150 g butter. International demand exists. However, to meet this demand, most Malian shea has to transit through the Republic of Côte d'Ivoire or Burkina Faso. The exporters we spoke to confirmed this practice, citing Holland and India as their main customers. An interesting study by CECI on the brand image of shea in 2007 provides information on Malian consumption of shea. It is the result of a survey with a sample size of 500 urban dwellers (in Bamako and Sikasso). The profile of the Malian consumer identified by this study corresponds to the married 21-40 age group. This group accounts for 58.8% of consumers. As for the form of the products consumed, the tables below show how, provide information on the nature and frequency of use.

Table 4: Use of shea products in Mali, 2007

Shea butter product	Percentage
Raw butter for moisturising	99,20
Raw butter for cooking oil	97,40
Moisturising cream	87,60
Handcrafted soap	86,00
Industrial soap	66.00
Lip balm	18,20

Table 5: Frequency of use in Mali, 2007

Product Frequency	Often	Occasionally	Rarely	Never	Don't know
Raw hydration	55	30	9	7	0
Cooking	42	38	10	0	0
Moisturising cream	10	15	15	52	7
Hand-made soap	30	28	18	0	3
Industrial soap	11	7	5	60	18
Lip balm	23	32	13	8	8

The main reasons for using shea butter, in addition to its cosmetic properties, are

• For raw butter for moisturising, the medicinal properties are the most important;

• For raw butter for cooking, the food benefits are mentioned by 71.7% of users;

• 63.2% and 60% mention the cosmetic virtues of the moisturising cream and industrial soap respectively;

• For 80.7% of respondents, a key characteristic of handmade soap is its medicinal rather than cosmetic properties (7.8%).

• 62.4% of Malian consumers rank the medicinal properties of shea butter lip balm ahead of its cosmetic properties (36.2%).

The survey also revealed that 89.4% of Malian consumers, once well informed about the concept of fair trade, were prepared to buy these products, even though the prices were higher (2007) [37].

c) Commercial circuit

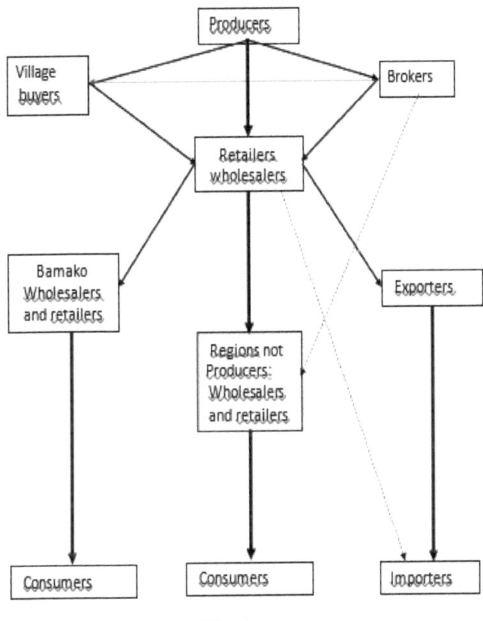

Captions:

Very common Common Common Rare

***Figure 3**: Shea butter marketing network in Mali, including cooperatives [37].*

1.2.7. Cosmetic and pharmaceutical uses of shea butter

Although shea butter has been used for thousands of years in Africa, it is now a highly prized raw material for industry. It is used in the food industry and above all in the cosmetics and pharmaceutical industries.

a) Use in cosmetology

Although limited in relation to the needs of the food industry, demand for shea butter in the cosmetics industry is relatively high. As with all vegetable fats, the presence offree fatty acids and triglycerides in shea butter means it can be used in the formulation of cosmetic soaps, creams, milks and ointments. In addition, because of its high unsaponifiable matter content, it is said to have skin and hair repair and maintenance properties. In this respect, it is often used as agents :

✎ Capillary protection, thanks to the presence of vitamin A, which restores suppleness and vitality to damaged hair;

✎ For face and body care, because it moisturises and nourishes the surface layers of the skin,

protects it from the sun's UV rays and improves its elasticity by regenerating dead cells;
↳ Relaxing massages;

↳ Protection against the elements (cold, wind);

Shea butter can be found in cosmetic products [39] such as :
- Baby care products (5-8%) ;
- Hand creams (5-10%);
- Lip care (5-10%);
- Night care creams (8 to 15%);
- Products for dry and sensitive skin (5 to 12%);
- Products to prevent stretch marks during pregnancy (6-8%);
- Day creams (4 to 6%);
- Soaps (2 to 3%);
- Toothpastes (1%) ;
- Face masks (5%), etc... [5]

b) Use in pharmacies

Shea butter's unsaponifiable nature gives it anti-inflammatory and healing properties, which are used for massages and to treat aches and pains and head colds. These properties are also used in certain products to treat rheumatic pain and burns. Shea butter is also used as a fatty excipient in the preparation of ointments, milks and dermatological creams [39]. It can be found, for example, in analgesic preparations (Baume saint Bernard, hydrocortisone cream) and anti-acne preparations, in liniments and ointments.

2. Emulsions

2.1. Definitions

An emulsion is defined as a system in which a liquid is dispersed in fine droplets in another liquid. The two liquids must be immiscible. The liquid dispersed in the form of fine droplets is called the dispersed (or discontinuous) phase, while the other liquid in which the droplets diffuse is called the continuous (or dispersing) phase. Emulsions are therefore dispersed systems [52].

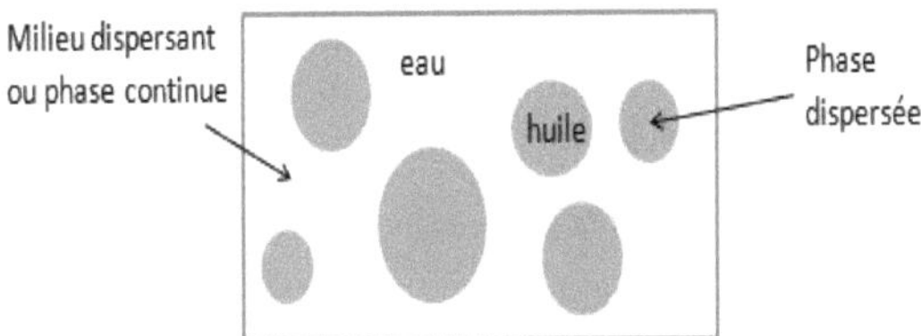

Figure 4: Phase diagram

Emulsions are found in many fields, including food, cosmetics, pharmaceuticals and petroleum, etc. This can be explained by the different types of emulsions that can be found [41] :

- Natural" emulsions such as milk, vinaigrette ..;
- Emulsions formed temporarily during certain stages of industrial processes (liquid-liquid extraction, emulsion polymerisation);
- Unwanted emulsions are formed during certain processes that we try to break, for example during the exploitation of oil fields. This phenomenon is also encountered in machining processes, degreasing and de-oiling waste water before discharge;
- The most commonly encountered formulated emulsions are

They can be used in a wide range of applications because they are easy to form, but also because of their many textures: fluid, creamy, jelly-like, etc., which explains their great interest in cosmetics (hygiene and beauty) and the food industry.

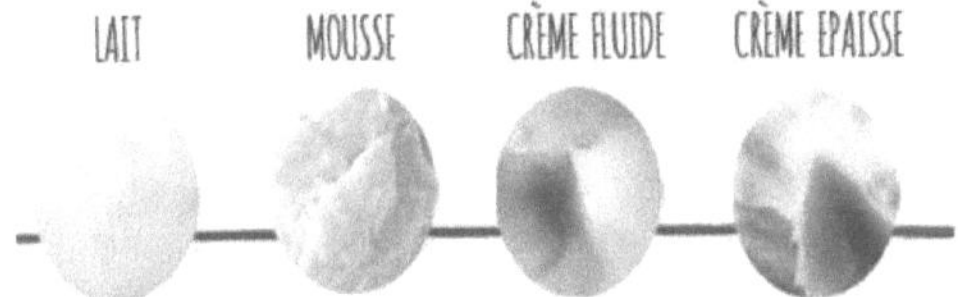

Figure 5: Different types of emulsion texture

2.2. The different types of emulsion

An emulsion is usually made up of two phases: a hydrophilic phase called water (E) and a lipophilic phase called oil (H).

- The hydrophilic phase |E|, also known as the aqueous phase, contains water and water-soluble compounds.
- The lipophilic phase |H|, also known as the fatty phase, oily phase or organic phase, is made up of a mixture of ingredients of various origins. It may be composed of oils, fats and/or waxes which, at room temperature, are in liquid, semi-solid and solid form respectively. Synthetic substances may also be used [40].

2.2.1. Simple emulsions

According to the pharmacopoeia, there are 2 forms of simple emulsion:

- Direct emulsions: O/W oil-in-water emulsions in which the

oil droplets are dispersed in water.

- Reverse emulsions: water-in-oil emulsions, W/O [40].

2.2.2. Double emulsions

Double emulsions are those simultaneously comprising O/W and W/O emulsions leading to either water-in-oil-in-water (W/O/W) or oil-in-water-in-oil (O/W/O) emulsions. Each globule dispersed in the double emulsion forms a vesicular structure containing single or multiple aqueous compartments separated from the second aqueous phase by an oil phase [40].

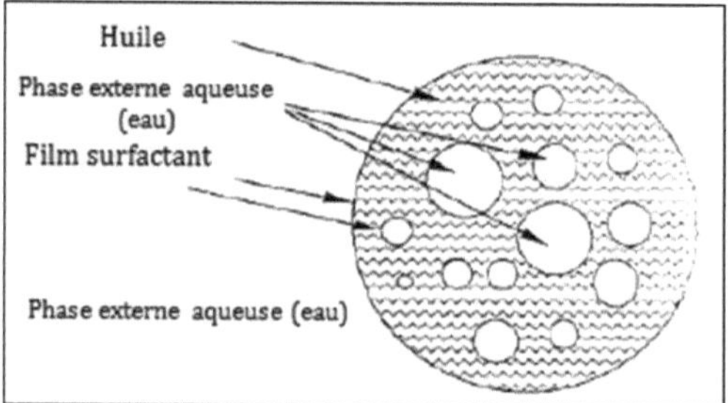

Figure 6: Diagram of a double W/O/W emulsion

As with single emulsions, there are 2 types of double emulsion:

- Water-in-oil-in-water (W/O/W) emulsions, in which a W/O emulsion is dispersed in the form of droplets in an aqueous phase. The oil droplets are surrounded by an aqueous phase, which in turn surrounds one or more water droplets. Their manufacture requires two surfactants: one hydrophobic to stabilise the interface of the internal W/O emulsion and one hydrophilic to stabilise the external interface of the oil globules.

- Oil-in-water-in-oil (O/W/O) emulsions, in which an O/W emulsion is dispersed in an oil phase. In this system

In an emulsion, the aqueous (hydrophilic) phase separates the internal and external oily phases. Water-in-oil-in-water (W/O/W) emulsions are the most common type of emulsion. used because they have broader application areas [42].

2.3. Surface tension and surfactants

a. Surface tension

As an emulsion is made up of 2 immiscible phases, the molecules at the liquid interface are not surrounded by molecules of the same nature, so they are not in equilibrium. A force therefore develops at the interface, which contracts the contact surface in order to stabilise the interface. This force is called interfacial tension. It exists at any interface between two different media (two solids, two liquids, or between a liquid and a solid). It can also be defined either as energy per unit area, or as a force per unit length. The unit of measurement for surface tension is the newton per metre (N/m) or J/m2. The higher the surface tension, the greater the energy required to produce the surface, and therefore the more difficult it will be to generate a drop.

b. Surfactants

Surfactants are amphiphilic molecules with a hydrophilic and a lipophilic part. The hydrophilic head forms hydrogen and ionic bonds with the hydrophilic phase, while the tail forms Van der Waals bonds and hydrophobic interactions with the lipophilic phase.

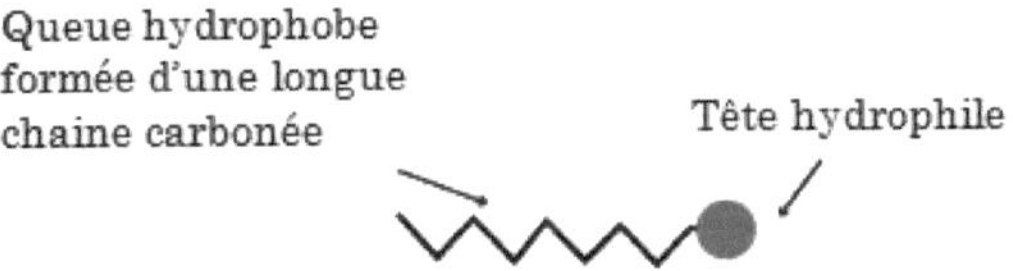

Figure 7: Simplified diagram of a surfactant

They have 3 important properties in terms of the manufacture and stability of emulsions:

- They reduce surface tension, which facilitates droplet formation and prevents immediate recombination of the droplet.

- They reduce the pressure gradient at the interface, which has the following effects stabilises droplets by repelling them from each other

- They stabilise the drops by preventing them from interacting with each other

The HLB (Hydrophilic-Lipophilic Balance) was developed by William C. Griffin in 1949. It is used to estimate the hydrophilic/lipophilic ratio and, above all, to choose a surfactant according to the direction of the chosen emulsion. The scale ranges from 1 to 20. The HLB value is high when the hydrophilic fraction is predominant and, conversely, it is low if the molecule is more lipophilic than hydrophilic. Knowing the HLB makes it easier to choose the surfactant at the time of use. The following table shows the different roles that surfactants can play depending on their HLB.

Table IVI: Role of surfactants as a function of HLB

HBL value	Role
3 à 6	W/O emulsifiers
8 à 18	O/W emulsifiers

Above a certain surfactant concentration called the critical micellar concentration (CMC), surfactants tend to form agglomerates called micelles. In water, the lipophilic ends of the surfactant face the inside of the micelle, while the hydrophobic ends form the interface between the micelle and the solvent. In an organic solvent, such as oil, the arrangement is reversed.

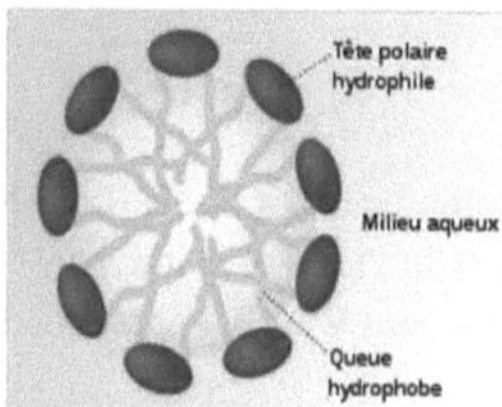

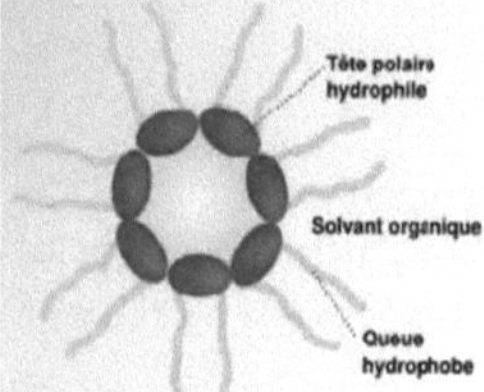

Figure 8: Diagram of a micelle. a- direct micelle; b- reverse micelle

In the presence of the two immiscible phases, the surfactant absorbs at the liquid-liquid interface and thus modifies the surface tension. The surface tension will decrease until it reaches a minimum value, which it will maintain despite a low concentration of surfactant (CMC): the surfactant is no longer concentrated enough to form micelles and fill the entire surface of the liquid.

2.4. Stability of emulsions

By definition, an emulsion is not a system at thermodynamic equilibrium (equality of chemical potentials between the two phases). The main phenomena responsible for the instability of emulsions are summarised below:

Table VII: Phenomena and causes of emulsion instability

Phenomena	Causes
Murissement d'Ostwald	Solubility of the dispersed phase in the dispersing phase
Creaming and sedimentation	Difference in density between the 2 phases
Flocculation	Repulsions insufficient between the droplets
Coalescence	Droplets come together and break up interfacial thread

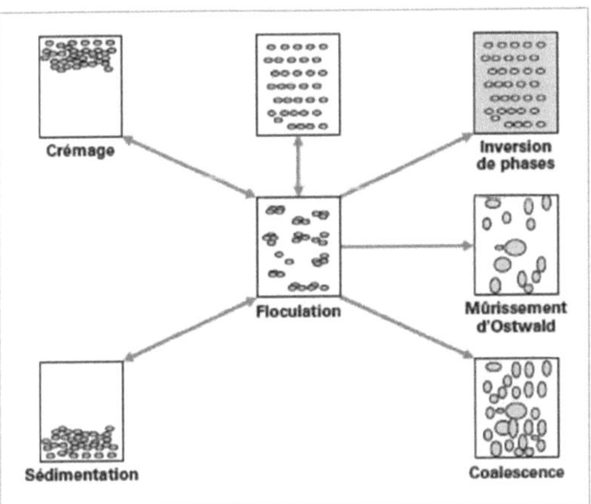

Figure 9: Phenomena involved in the destabilisation of emulsions [40].

2.4.1. Murissement d'Ostwald

This is known as ripening, as the smaller droplets diffuse into the larger ones through the continuous phase.

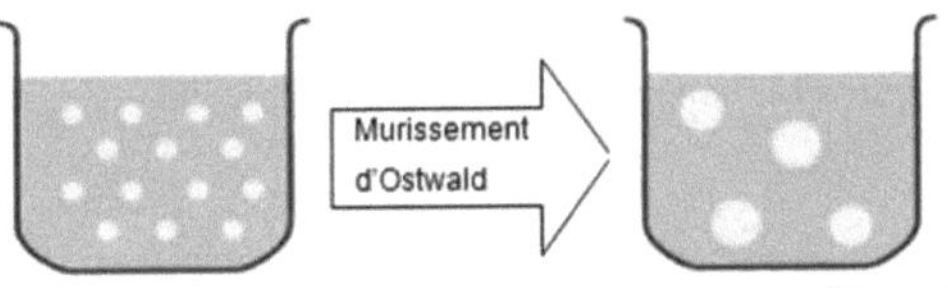

Figure 10: Murissement d'Ostwald

This phenomenon is due to the pressure difference inside the droplets and more specifically to the Laplace pressure exerted at the droplet interface. This represents the pressure difference between the convex and concave phases of the drop.

$$P_L = \frac{2y}{r}$$

With PL Laplace pressure (Pa) y interfacial tension (N/m) r main radius of curvature of the drop Laplace pressure is therefore proportional to interfacial tension and inversely proportional to drop size. It is very high for small drops and low for larger drops. Small drops are therefore difficult to fragment, which is why they diffuse into larger drops. For droplets between 50 and 200 nm, Ostwald ripening is the main destabilisation mechanism. When it starts to occur, it is almost impossible to stop because it tends to reduce the energy by minimising the interfacial surface [43].

This phenomenon can be controlled by :

- Homogenisation of droplet size;
- It can be delayed or interrupted by the addition of components that are poor or insoluble in the continuous phase.

2.4.2. Creaming and sedimentation [40]

The origin of these two phenomena lies in a difference in density between the dispersed and dispersing phases.In the creaming phenomenon, the droplets will migrate upwards from the dispersed phase (O/W emulsion), whereas in the sedimentation phenomenon they will migrate downwards (W/O emulsion). The size of the droplets, the difference in density between the two phases and gravity are the parameters that influence droplet migration. Creaming takes place if the density of the dispersed phase is greater than that of the dispersing phase, otherwise sedimentation occurs.

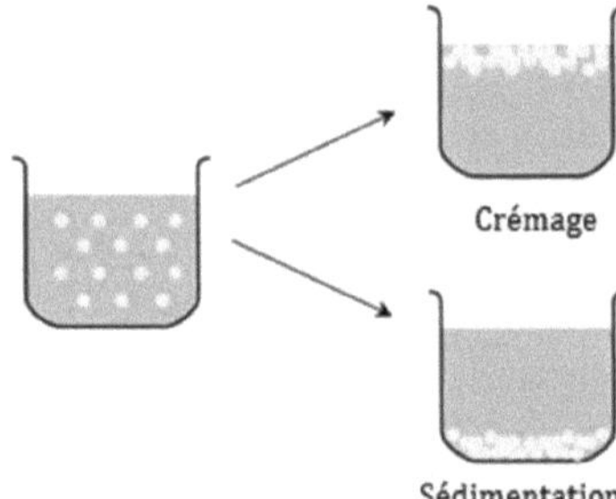

Figure 11: Creaming and sedimentation phenomena

These two phenomena can be controlled by increasing the viscosity of the dispersing phase or by using a texturising agent. They are also reversible: if the emulsion is reacted, it returns to its initial appearance. Over the long term, these phenomena concentrate the drops locally and accelerate instabilities such as coalescence.

2.4.3. Flocculation [40]

Flocculation begins in emulsions as soon as agitation is stopped. Aggregates begin to form very quickly: their formation time ranges from a few fractions of a second to several seconds, depending on the concentration of the internal aqueous phase. However, their structure in E/H emulsions and the speed of their formation depend on the concentration of the dispersed phase.

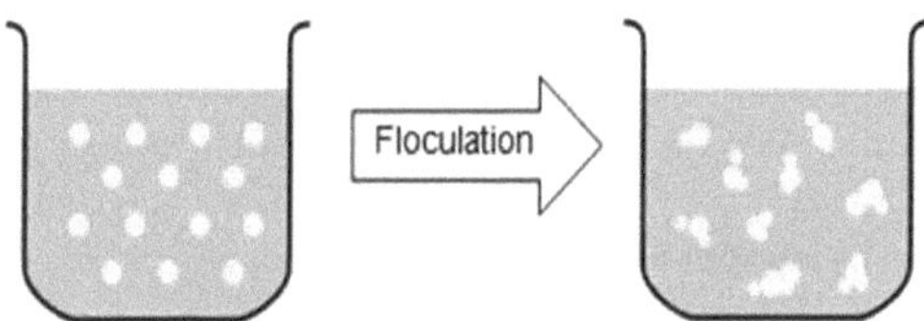

Figure 12: Flocculation phenomenon

For aqueous droplets between 100 and 300 nm in size, Brownian motion is the main reason for flocculation. If particles collide, this leads to the formation of aggregates containing hundreds of droplets. These aggregates can have a compact spherical shape. In this case, an increase in the size of the aggregates leads to their sedimentation and the separation of the organic phase from the emulsion. Furthermore, these aggregates can be branched structures which occupy almost the entire volume of the O/W or W/O emulsions [44]. However, flocculation can be controlled:

- By increasing the viscosity of the dispersing phase, because a thicker dispersing phase reduces the speed of collision between droplets;
- By adding surfactants

It is also a reversible phenomenon: agitation allows the drops to be resuspended.

2.4.4. Coalescence

Coalescence occurs when there is a break in the protective film of the continuous phase. This is due to the droplets coming together, which will tend to reduce the thin film under the effect of the pressure exerted on the droplets. The droplets will then merge to form larger droplets. Eventually, the emulsion may break up or go out of phase.

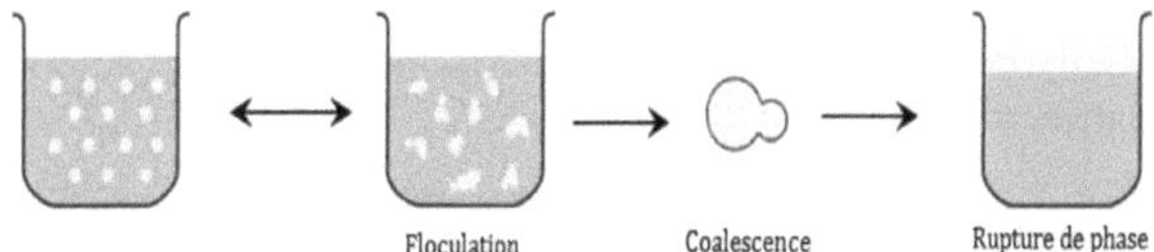

Figure 13: Coalescence or phase break-up phenomenon

To limit this phenomenon, it is preferable to use a surfactant that will reinforce the protective film by increasing interfacial elasticity.

2.5. Batch processes for preparing emulsions

The manufacture of emulsions requires an external energy input which is the Most often mechanical, but can also be sonic, electrical or other.Emulsification processes are usually classified according to the mechanism involved. There are 2 main categories [45]:

- Those that generate shear: these mainly include moving parts specifically designed for emulsification (turbines and propellers), rotor-stator devices and colloidal mills;

- Processes involving cavitation, such as ultrasonic techniques and high-pressure homogenisers.

2.5.1. Emulsification by mechanical agitation

a) Manufacturing stages

The different stages in the manufacture of an emulsion are shown in the figure below:

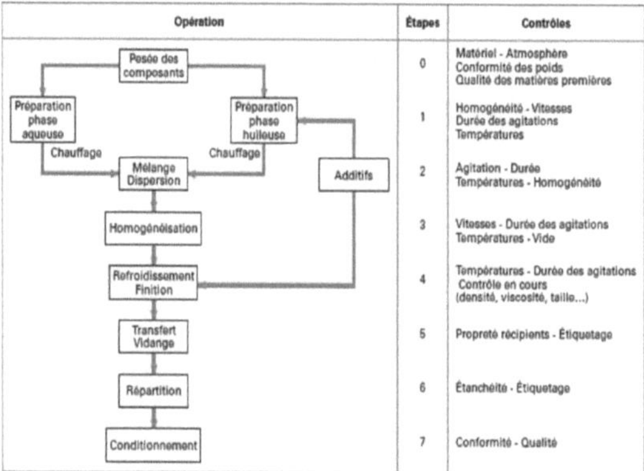

Figure 14: Stages in the manufacture of an emulsion [45].

There are 2 main successive stages [45] :

- A pre-emulsification stage: this involves suspending droplets of the dispersed phase in the continuous phase (dispersion-mixing stage). In most cases, the phase to be dispersed is introduced gradually into the continuous phase where mechanical agitation is applied. This will produce droplets approximately 100 μm in size;

- A homogenisation stage: as the drops generated in the first stage are too large, the aim here is to reduce their size in order to stabilise the emulsion.

The dispersion system chosen must cause sufficiently high shear to ensure good dispersion, circulation and liquid transport so that the entire volume can pass through the dispersion zone in a given time or transit time [41-45].

b) Dispersers

The main objective of dispersers is to ensure good shear in order to encourage droplet break-up. Circulation is also an important parameter to take into account, as it influences the size distribution. As the drops move away from the agitator and therefore from the shear zone, they tend to coalesce. Turbines such as Rushton-type turbines or turbines with inclined blades generating high shear are preferred. The drops produced will be between 10 and 100 µm in size [45].

c) Homogenisers

Homogenisers are used to obtain the desired particle size and good stability. To achieve this, the mobiles used have a high shear rate. The most commonly used is the rotor-stator system, where the liquid is sucked into the working head, passes through the rotor and stator blades where it undergoes high shear before being expelled and re-emerging. The droplets produced are relatively small, in the micrometre range. This is why these systems are used directly or after a pre-emulsification stage [45].

2.5.2. Static mixer

A static mixer consists of a set of immobile elements placed end-to-end in a tube. Each element has a particular rigid geometric structure that divides the flow and recombines it. Generally, the fluids are brought into contact by the radial movement taking place in the mixers, and they circulate with the aid of a pump. This system has a homogeneous shear and particle size distribution, resulting in relatively fine emulsions (of the order of 1 µm in diameter) [45].

2.5.3. Phase reversal

This is the transformation of an O/W emulsion into a W/O emulsion or vice versa. There are a number of possible mechanisms behind this phenomenon:

- A change in temperature ;

- A change in composition: for example, if an aqueous phase containing a hydrophilic surfactant is added to an oily phase containing a lipophilic surfactant, or by adding a large volume of the initially dispersed phase.

2.5.4. Membrane emulsification

This is a relatively recent method that has developed enormously over the last fifteen years. It is a very interesting technique given its low energy consumption and excellent control of droplet size and size distribution. We have seen that single emulsions can be prepared under high shear conditions in order to obtain small droplets (for example, by mechanical agitation). Double emulsions, on the other hand, are made with lower shear to avoid breaking the internal droplets [46]. Indeed, high shear would cause internal diffusion in the droplets, which would increase the frequency of collisions, and therefore the coalescence of the internal droplets with the external aqueous phase [47].

As shear stresses are gentle during membrane emulsification, this is an interesting process for their manufacture. Double emulsions are prepared by emulsifying single emulsions with an excess of aqueous or oily phase, depending on whether they are W/O/W or O/W/O, respectively.Two operating modes are used: membrane emulsification with cross-flow and membrane pre-mixing.

a) Cross-flow membrane emulsification

In this operating mode, the primary emulsion is formed by membrane emulsification. The phase to be dispersed is pressed through a microporous membrane while the continuous phase flows along the surface of the membrane. Droplets form through the pores. They break off when they reach a critical size. When the pores are not cylindrical, an important force comes into play: the force resulting from the deformation of the phase to be dispersed in the pore. This force can become dominant in certain cases. This method is used to fix the size of the drops, which will be larger than the smallest of the pore radii.

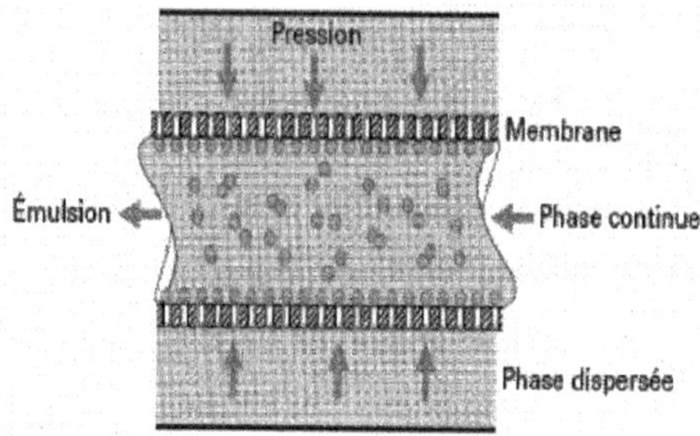

Figure 15: Schematic representation of a simple cross-flow emulsification process

The solution containing the simple emulsion is then pressed through the membrane pores, thus forming the double emulsion [48].

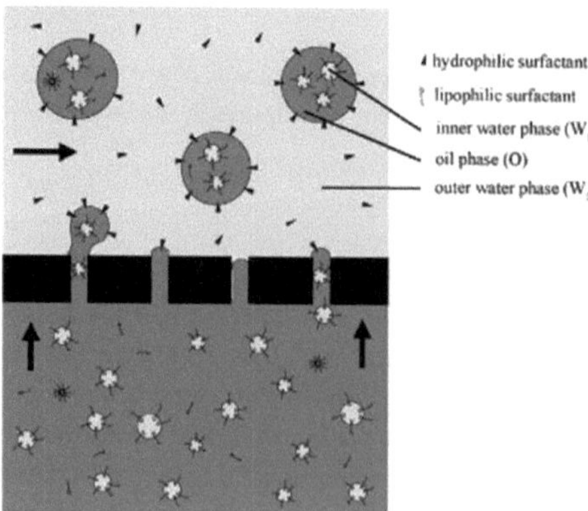

Figure 16: Schematic representation of a double cross-flow emulsification process

b) Membrane pre-mix

An initial coarse premix is produced comprising simple emulsions. It is then pushed through a membrane. After the large droplets have passed through this membrane, the droplets break down into droplets and are doubled. The droplet size distribution obtained is slightly wider than those obtained with the cross-flow membrane emulsification method.

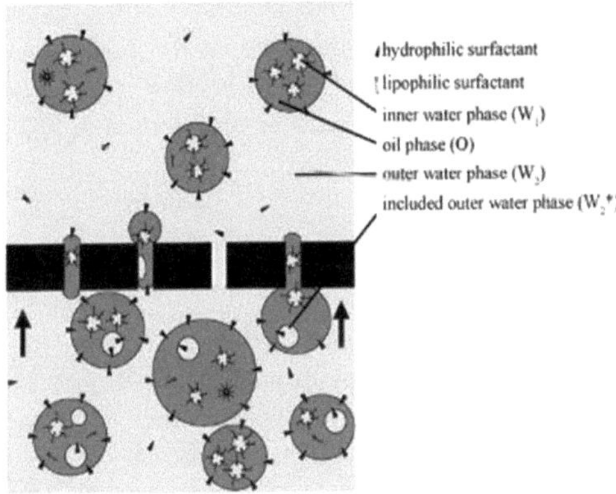

Figure 17: Schematic representation of double emulsification by membrane pre-mixing

For these two formation mechanisms, it is very important that the membrane remains constantly wetted by the continuous phase so that the droplets form and separate properly. A notable disadvantage of this technique is the low flux of the dispersed phase caused by the low hydraulic permeability of most of the membranes used. However, the flux of the dispersed phase can be increased by using a membrane with low hydraulic resistance [8].

2.5.5. Other techniques

a) Cross-flow membrane emulsification with SPG membranes Mine et al. were the first to report the possibility of producing double emulsions (W/O/W) by membrane emulsification with Shirasu porous glass (SPG). They used a microfluidiser for the first W/O emulsion and SPG membranes to produce the double emulsion. They found that the membrane must be hydrophilic. In addition, it must have an average pore size of at least twice the diameter of the water droplets in the primary W/O emulsion. If this is not the case, the droplets will be rejected by the membrane. Furthermore, the concentration of internal water droplets for the manufacture of W/O/W emulsions must be between 30 and 50% by volume. However, Okochi and Nakano obtained good results with a lower proportion [48]. This is a reliable and reproducible method for producing stable emulsions. whenever surfactants are used.A disadvantage of this method compared with conventional methods is the long time it takes to produce emulsions due to the low flow rates. This could be a problem if the stability of the active ingredients used is low.

b) Microchannel emulsification

This is a new process used to produce monodisperse emulsions. The droplets obtained are much more monodisperse than those obtained by mechanical agitation or membrane emulsification.In this process, small non-cylindrical microchannels are formed in a silicon wafer. Droplets are produced by forcing the dispersed phase through the microchannels. This technique therefore uses interfacial tension, the advantages of the micrometric scale and the forceto form the droplets. This process is interesting for the production of double emulsions because the droplets are formed via the low shear flow of the continuous phase.One disadvantage of this method, which still needs to be improved, is its low emulsion production rate [48].

2.5.6. Disadvantages of these manufacturing processes

a. Energy aspect

In order to produce emulsions, the systems mentioned above, particularly those requiring mechanical agitation, are very energy-intensive. This is mainly due to the energy supplied by the turbine and the shear required to break up the droplets. This energy is transmitted by the dispersion system and is divided into viscous dissipation within the liquid, dissipated energy used for fragmentation and interfacial energy. Shear will dissipate a large part of the energy supplied by the turbine. The mechanical energy will be dissipated in the form of heat, hence the importance of cooling the formulation during emulsification in order to control the temperature. We could also mention Laplace pressure, which, like interfacial energy, is present at the interfaces, and represents part of the energy to be supplied to our system [41]. It should be noted that the energy consumption of a mobile is related to the type of flow it implements in the tank [45]. Temperature is also an important parameter because it will influence the quality of the emulsion. Temperature can affect the viscosity of the medium but can also modify the interfacial free energy [41].

b. Size of emulsions

In general, in an emulsion, the droplets of the dispersed phase are not of a single size. This is why we talk about particle size distribution. This parameter is important because it has an impact on the stability of the emulsion (particularly ripening). It is well established that mechanical processes result in a wide size distribution. Microfluidics, on the other hand, seems to produce monodisperse emulsions.

2.6. Continuous emulsion manufacturing processes

A great deal of progress has been made since 1990 in terms of processes and understanding of physico-chemical phenomena. It is therefore possible to design new operating methods based on new production methods or scales. The primary objective here is to produce with reduced energy consumption, in smaller volumes, with greater efficiency and minimising environmental impact by using fewer solvents, for example, by reducing the number of production stages [49]. In some cases, this can involve microtechnologies such as microfluidics, which use continuous processes. The manufacturing method used in this thesis is developed in the experimental section.Continuously operating process systems have a number of advantages, such as lower energy consumption and uniform, controlled size distribution, which is not the case with discontinuous systems. However, the implementation of the continuous process is much more cumbersome than that of the batch process. This is because the pump system needs to be adapted to the viscosity of the products, as well as the flow control systems. These systems are not yet widespread, but they have great potential.

PART I

METHODOLOGY

I. Location and type of study

I.1. Place of study

Our study took place at the Hospital Pharmacy of the Hôpital de Dermatology Unit in Bamako.

a. Bamako Dermatology Hospital (HDB)

Located in the Djicoroni para district of Bamako, the Bamako Dermatology Hospital was created by order n° 2019-010 of 27 March 2019, ratified by the law of 23 July 2019. Its organisation and operating procedures were laid down by decree N^0 2019-0246/P-RM of 27 March 2019. The hospital's mission is to diagnose and treat skin diseases and dermatological problems resulting from sexually transmitted infections and other dermatological conditions, and to deal with dermatological emergencies and referrals. It must also participate in continuing university education and promote research.

b. The hospital pharmacy at the Bamako Dermatology Hospital

The hospital pharmacy is one of the hospital's departments. This is subdivided into several compartments:

- The sales area ;
- The shop;
- The free space ;
- Galenic unit ;
- The head of department's office.

I.2. Type of study

This is an experimental descriptive study.

II. Materials and methods

II.1. Equipment

II.1.1. Description of equipment and small laboratory materials

The following equipment and small laboratory materials were used:

- **Beaker**

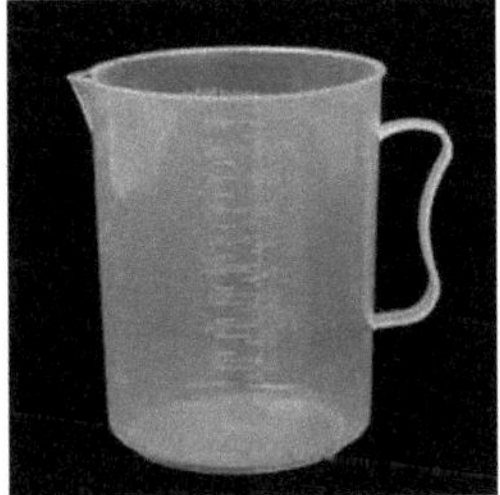

Figure 18 : 1000 ml transparent plastic beaker with handle

- **Balance**

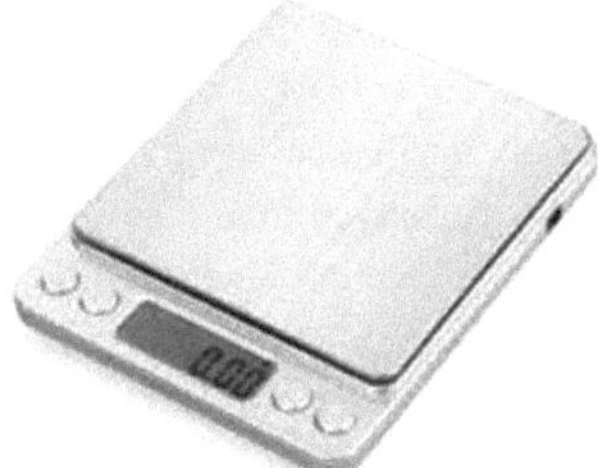

Figure 19: Beautymix precision balance Model: BM01 (MF03-1)

- **Timer**

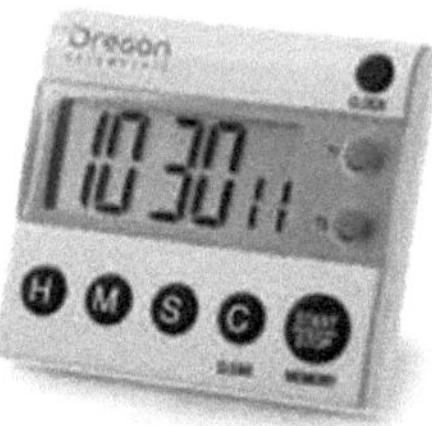

Figure 20: Digital quartz laboratory timer

Electric work table

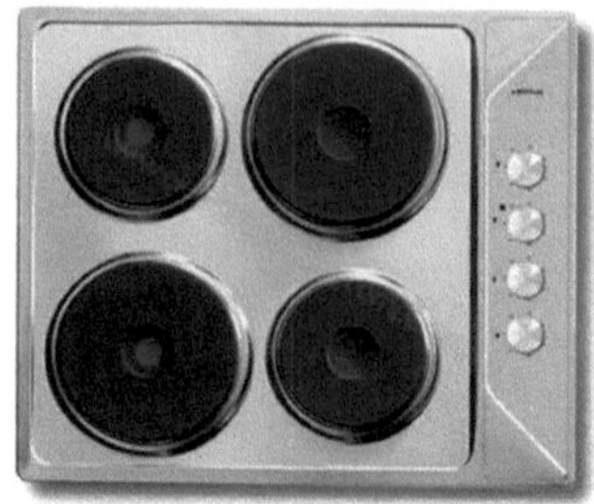

Specification Type 15023 B
Power supply: 220 V 220v 50 hz 6000W
Figure 21: AILUX AIRDIS electric work table

➯ Water distiller

Description

Specifications and special features Tankless benchtop mono-distiller. Excellent distillate quality, conductivity approx. 2.3 us/cm at 25°C (see technical data). Thermostatic dry-run protection. Energy saving through distillation of preheated cooling water. Boiler easily accessible for cleaning. Distillate is discharged from the condenser via a hose. CO2 degassing via condenser. Refrigerant water temperature indicated by thermometer. Stainless steel heating element, boiler and condenser. Electrolytically zinced sheet metal casing with electrostatic epoxy powder coating. Water inlet and outlet connections ½ inch (ø approx. 12.7 mm) Water inlet and outlet hoses available as an option. Range of applications GFL distilled water units are used in research and development for bacteriological and clinical sample preparation, as well as for cell and tissue culture preparation and for the formulation of reagents and ointments. The distillate is also used for cleaning and sterilisation, for buffer solutions and for microbiological and analytical applications.

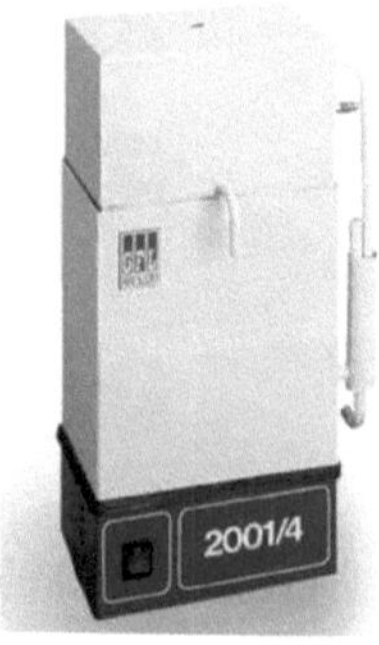

Figure 21: Water distiller 2001/4

✧ Mixing agitator

Description

Digital aerial laboratory shaker

Apply to a stable liquid stirrer, particularly for mixing a small quantity of water. volume of oil, chemical and medical samples. It has been specially designed for health applications, environment, biochemical experiments, education and scientific research. The LCD display shows the set speed and actual value, and real-time monitoring of speed and time.
Can precisely control stirring speed, with a speed range of 200 to 3000 rpm.

Overload protection, loop protection, soft start, prevents overflow.
Model specification: 20 l
Motor power: 200 W Chuck torque: 90 N.CM Power supply: 220 V
Speed range: 200 to 3000 rpm

Max. stirring volume (H2O): 0 ~ 20 l

Stirring speed display: digital LCD display Resolution: +/- 1 rpm
Stirring rod length: 300 mm

Stirring rod material: 304 stainless steel Chuck range: Ø0.5-10
Product dimensions: 200 x 315 x 600 mm Gross weight: 10 kg
Permitted environment: 40-105° F, 80% RH Max. viscosity: **10,000 (mPa.s); 80,000 (mPa.s)**

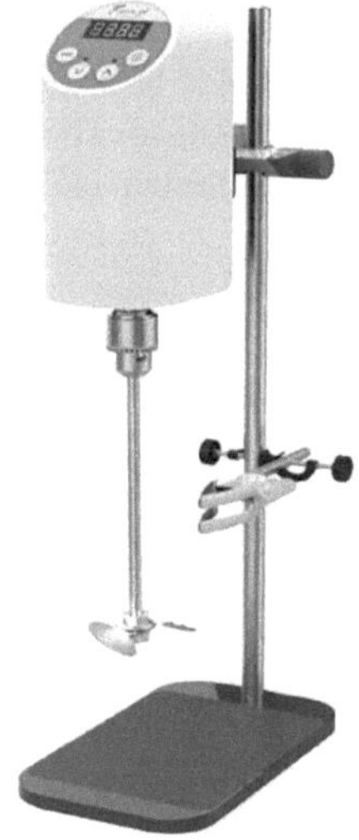

Figure 22: YUEWO Lab Digital electric Shaker Mixer

II.1.2. Raw materials

The raw materials are listed in the table below.

Table VIII: Raw materials and suppliers

Name	Roles	Area of origin / suppliers
Shea butter	Fats	COPROKAZAN-Bougouni Email :ugfz@coprokazan.org Tel : (+223) 69 12 66 43
Distilled water	Excipient ; aqueous vehicle	HDB Laboratory

* We chose this butter over another because it had a certificate of conformity. and a laboratory test report attesting to its purity.

II.2. Methods

II.2.1. Qualitative and quantitative cream formulations

II.2.1.1. Qualitative formulations

For the choice of butter, we looked for a butter that could guarantee a certain purity and therefore had to have passed certain laboratory tests. The water had to be distilled and therefore pathogen-free. What's more, it had to be used at room temperature, because hot or cold preparation does not give conclusive results. For the packaging, we asked for transparent glass jars in order to assess the behaviour of the formulations during the experimental process. The packaging had to have a plastic cap to avoid any risk of corrosion and therefore contamination of the formulation. The balance had to be right, and the agitator had to have a capacity of at least 1200 rpm.

II.2.1.2. Quantitative formulations

We used a one-dimensional shea butter scanning method to determine the correct proportions of butter needed to form stable emulsions with water without the addition of any stabilising agent. The quantities of water ranged from 0 to 90% in the formulas with scales of ten (10) to 10. In addition, all the tests were carried out three (03) times in order to confirm the results obtained. The table below shows the composition of the formulas studied.

Table IX: Quantitative composition (g) of emulsions

Formulas	Shea butter	Distilled water
1	100	0
2	90	10
3	80	20
4	70	30
5	60	40
6	50	50
7	40	60
8	30	70
9	20	80
10	10	90

*These are the formulas used to make the creams shown in Figures 28 and 29.

II.2.1.2. Manufacturing process

The creams were prepared using the indirect emulsification method. The equipment used for preparation was washed, dried and sterilised beforehand. The aqueous phase (distilled water) was introduced into a 1000 ml plastic beaker and the external oily phase (shea butter) was placed in a water bath with its original container for approximately 35 minutes to be liquefied. We then removed the butter from the water bath and placed it on the bench. We then waited 3 minutes for it to reach a temperature of around 65°C. We then proceeded to the actual emulsification. To do this, we placed an empty beaker on the balance and tared it. Using a spatula, we removed the quantity of shea butter needed for the formula and placed it in the beaker. Then we tared it again and added the amount of distilled water needed for the formula. The whole mixture was then placed under a YUEWO propeller shaker for 6 minutes (with the stopwatch running). Once the 6 minutes had elapsed, we stopped the stirrer when the stopwatch sounded and switched on the balance. We then weighed the whole formula again to determine the losses and compensate for them by adding corresponding quantities of distilled water.Finally, we emptied the contents of the beaker into the glass jars, placed them on the bench and waited for at least 2 hours. Formulas that did not produce an emulsion with a homogeneous appearance after cooling to room temperature were eliminated from the tests.

II.2.1.3. Cream packaging

The creams were packaged in 100 g clear glass jars as shown in figure 27. This type of packaging has no influence on the stability of the emulsions [4]. The creams were stored at room temperature on the laboratory bench. The jars were labelled with the formula number ending with the triplicate number. Example: (1-1); (1-2); (1-3); ...

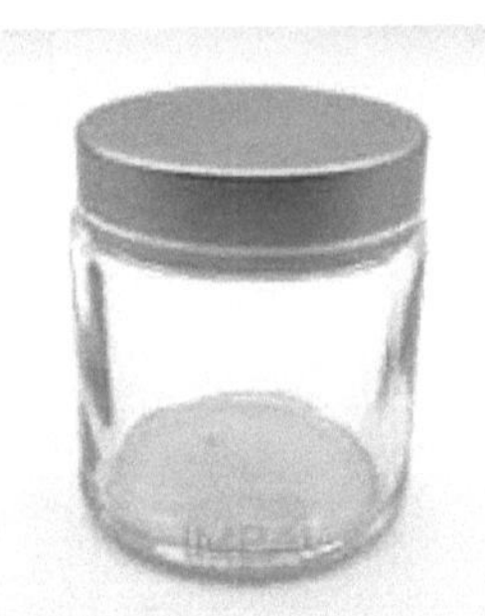

Figure 23: Glass packaging

In the next stage we checked the physical stability of the creams that had been formulated. The aim was to identify a range of stability allowing define the optimum quantities of butter needed to stabilise emulsions over time.

II.2.2. Evaluation of the influence of the percentage of shea butter on the physical stability and texture of emulsions

The tests were carried out on emulsions that showed a homogeneous appearance after cooling to room temperature (minimum 2h after the end of the manufacturing process). All tests were triplicated to confirm the repeatability of the experiment.

II.2.2.1. Control of the stability and fineness of emulsion droplets

II.2.2.1.1. Macroscopic appearance

It was used to observe the visual appearance of the preparations with the naked eye. It gave an indication of the particle size of the droplets, as shown in table (X) below:

Table X: Appearance of emulsions according to globule size [51].

Size of globules	Types of emulsion	Appearance macroscopic
> 5 µm	Coarse emulsions ± stable	Milky white
5 to 1 µm	Medium emulsions	Milky white
1 µm to 0.5 µm	Fine emulsions	White + bluish sheen
0.5 µm to 0.1 µm	Light emulsions translucent	Semi-transparent
< 0.1µm	Translucent microemulsions Micellar solutions	Transparent

II.2.2.1.2. Determining the direction of the emulsion :

The emulsion rinsing method: O/W emulsion rinses off easily with water, while the opposite is true for W/O emulsions. We spread the cream on the back of our hand and ran it under a jet of water from the tap.

II.2.2.1.3. Bottle Test or stability test in a test tube :

This test was carried out under ambient storage conditions for 3 months. It consisted of monitoring changes over time in the macroscopic appearance of the emulsions, such as colour and homogeneity (the appearance or non-appearance of creaming and/or sedimentation phenomena and phase separation). These different paramcters were evaluated at specific times **(D0, D3, D7, D15, D30, D60 and D90**).

II.2.3. Identification o f a stability range for water/butter emulsions from shea

After assessing the stability parameters, we determined a range within which the water/shea butter preparations give stable emulsions after 3 months' storage at room temperature.

PART II

RESULTS

I. FORMULATIONS AND PREPARATION OF CREAMS

Ten (10) creams were formulated (Table VII) At the end of preparation, creams one (01) to four (04) and eight (08) to ten (10) were fluid 2 hours after emulsification. While creams five (05) to seven (7) (07) were thick. The figure below shows the ten (10) creams 2 hours after production.

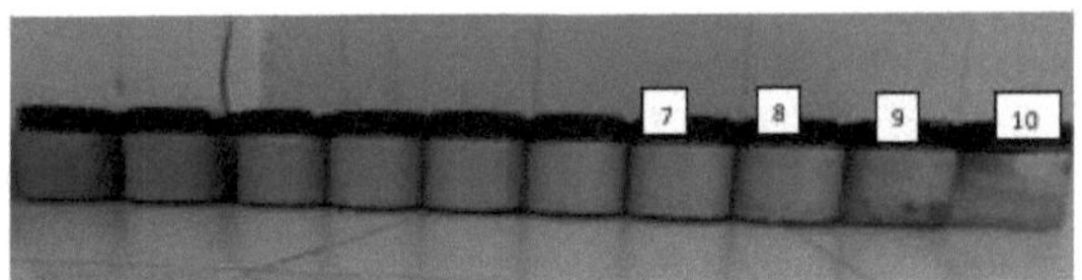

Figure 24: Creams 2h after production in the laboratory

Creams nine (09) and ten (10) were withdrawn from the tests because they were not stable 2 hours after formulation. Stability tests were carried out on creams one (01) to eight (08). The triplicates gave the same result each time. The figure below shows the eight (08) creams at D1.

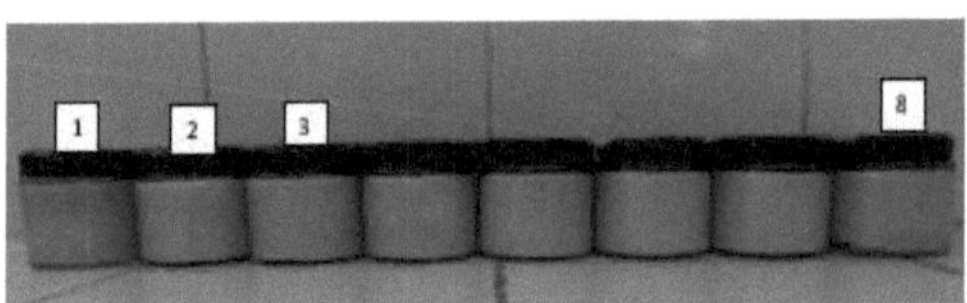

Figure 25: Creams at D1 after storage in the laboratory at room temperature

II. CREAM STABILITY

II .1. Macroscopic aspect

All the creams had a milky white appearance and were semi-solid to solid in consistency. We therefore deduce that the size of the globules was between one (01) and five (05) µm, which corresponds to an average emulsion.

II. 2. Direction of emulsion

Not all our emulsions were water-washable, they were W/O type.

II.3. Bottle test

The physical stability and fluidity of the creams improved from D0-D90 (Table IX).

Table VIII: Changes in fluidity and physical stability of creams from D0-D90

Creams	Observations 2h	Comments J1	Comments J3	Comments J7	Observations J15	Observations J30	Comments J60	Comments J 90
1	F++ S J++	E+ S J++	E+ S J++	E++ S J++	E+++ S J++	E+++ S J++	E+++ S J++	E+++ S J++
2	F++ S J++	E+ S J++	E+ S J++	E++ S J++	E+++ S J++	E+++ S J++	E+++ S J++	E+++ S J++
3	F+ S J+	E+ S J+	E++ S J+	E+++ S J+	E+++ S J+	E+++ S J+	E+++ S J+	E+++ S J+
4	F+ S J+	E+ S B+	E++ S B+	E++ S B+	E+++ S B+	E+++ S B+	E+++ S B+	E+++ S B+
5	E+ S B+	E+ S B++	E++ S B++	E++ S B++	E++ S B++	E++ S B+	E++ S B+	E++ S B+
6	E+ S B+	E++ S B++	E++ S B++	E++ S B++	E++ S B++	E++ S B++	E++ S B++	E++ S B++
7	E++ S B+	E+++ S B++	E+++ S B++	E+++ S B++	E+++ S B++	E+++ S B++	E+++ S B++	E+++ S B++
8	F+++ S B++	F++ S B++	E+ I B++	-	-	-	-	-
9	F+++ I B++	-	-	-	-	-	-	-
10	F+++ I B++	-	-	-	-	-	-	-

F=Fluid E=Thick S=Stable I=Unstable C=Colour (Yellow, White) Weak + Medium ++ Strong+++

Changes in fluidity: The appearance of the different creams developed differently over time. Creams one (01) to four (04) went from fluid to thick from D1 and continued to thicken over time. Creams five (05) to seven (07), which were already thick at the end of the manufacturing process (2 h after resting in the laboratory), continued to thicken. Cream eight (08) went from fluid and stable to thick and unstable at D3.

Evolution of physical instability: The first unstable creams were creams nine (09) and ten (10); observation made 2 h after resting in the laboratory. Then at D3, cream eight (08). The most stable creams after 90 days were one
(01) to sept (07).

Stability interval: the most stable creams were those from one (01) to seven (07) with a water content of between 0 and 60%. Shea butter can therefore incorporate up to 60% water without showing signs of instability after 90 days according to the manufacturing method described above.

PART III
COMMENTS AND DISCUSSIONS

I. Limits

This study investigated the emulsifying properties of Malian shea butter from the Bougouni region. The limitations of our study were that the microscopic aspect was not determined and it was difficult to carry out the centrifugation test, as the formulations obtained were very thick, even pasty. Furthermore, we were not sufficiently equipped to carry out more advanced research; analysing particle size in order to measure their granulometric distribution or determining the viscosity of the preparations obtained are all important tests that would have enabled us to take the research a little further if it had been possible to carry out laser diffraction or if we had had a penetrometer at our disposal.

II. Macroscopic appearance

The size of the globules is a very important parameter, as it makes it possible to predict the stability of the creams that have been formulated; the finer the globules, the more stable the cream is over a long period. In our study, all our emulsions had a milky white appearance, which corresponds to a medium emulsion or a coarse emulsion that is +/- stable. The globule size obtained for all our creams was therefore between one (01) and five (05) μm. This size guarantees average emulsion stability over the long term.

III. Direction of emulsion

The direction of the emulsion is a very important parameter which gives an indication of the stability of the preparations. In our study, all the preparations were W/O after a water washability test. This may be due to the indirect emulsification technique we used in slowly incorporating water into the oil phase. The indirect emulsification technique results in emulsions of the W/O type, where the oily phase is the continuous phase and the aqueous phase is the dispersed phase. We decided to use this technique rather than the classic direct emulsification technique, because it allows us to obtain creams that provide immediate comfort for the driest, most dehydrated skins by providing them with greater quantities of nutrition that is immediately accessible.

IV. Stability over time

IV.1. Changes in fluidity

Two (02) hours after preparing the creams, formulations one (01) to four (04) were fluid, while formulations five (05) to seven (07) went from fluid to slightly thick or even thick. Formula eight (08) remained very fluid. We noticed that the more diluted the formula, the faster it tended to solidify. This is due to the formulation process used; as the proportion of water in the formula increases, the cooling temperature of the butter is reached more quickly and so the formula crystallises more quickly. As shea butter is made up of ingredients that give it a non-negligible solid phase at room temperature, these ingredients cause emulsions to thicken (Tadros et al 2008). Finally, we observed an increase in the consistency of the creams over time (from D1 to D90) before finally stabilising after a more or less long period depending on the formulation. This could be explained by the fact that semi-solid or solid fats at room temperature, such as shea butter, tend to lead to an increase in texture over time. This increase is probably due to a reorganisation of the structure. of the preparations [2,4]. These results are identical to those obtained by Dr TOE [4].

IV.2. Evolution of physical instabilities

The emulsion must not demix. The first demixings were observed with the creams nine (09) and ten (10); 02 h after their preparation. They were therefore eliminated from the experimental process. Then, at D3, cream eight (08) also showed signs of demixing. At D90, creams one (01) to seven (07) were stable. These results can be explained by the fact that shea butter has a composition rich in fatty acids, in particular oleic acid (40 to 60%) and stearic acid (20 to 50%) [29,30], making them the major components of the butter. Oleic acid is used as an emulsifier in foods and topical pharmaceutical formulations [50]. In topical formulations, stearic acid is used as an emulsifier and solubilising agent [50].

IV.3. Evolution of the stability interval

The range of stability evolved over time from 70% at D3 to finally stabilise at 60% at D90. We can therefore conclude that shea butter can absorb up to 60% water and can therefore incorporate almost twice its weight in water without showing signs of instability, just like lanolin. This could be explained by its physical and chemical properties, in particular its stearic acid-rich composition. Partially neutralised stearic acid forms a creamy base when mixed with five (05) to fifteen (15) times its own weight of aqueous liquid [50].

CONCLUSION AND OUTLOOK

The aim of our work was to study the ability of a product to stabilise an emulsion.Composed largely of oleic and stearic acids, shea butter combined with water produces stable emulsions in well-defined proportions. This characteristic gives it emulsifying properties, so it can absorb almost twice its weight in water.However, it would be important to study the physico-chemical properties of Malian shea butter from the Bougouni region in order to complete this study.A study of the emulsifying and physico-chemical properties of shea butters from all over the shea belt in order to carry out comparative studies would provide definitive confirmation of this hypothesis.

REFERENCES

1. **Sanou H, Lamien N.** Vitellaria paradoxa: Shea. Saforgen 2017. ISBN: 978-84-694- 3165-8. Available at https://citarea.cita-aragon.es/citarea/bitstream/10532/1689/ 2/2011_342EN.pdf

2. **FAO,** and **OMS.** 2017. "REGIONAL STANDARD FOR UNREFINED SHEA BUTTER. CXS 325R Adopted In PDF Free Download." https://docplayer.fr/76427708-Norme-regionale-pour-le-beurre-de-karite-non-raffine-cxs-325r-adoptee-en-2017.html.

3. **Sanogo R**. Beurre De Karité En Dermopharmacie.ppt [Internet]. Presentation : Afephar fourth scientific day ; 2016 [cited 10 Oct 2017]; Bamako. Available from: www.cnop.sante.gov.ml/docs/BeurreDeKariteEnDermopharmacie.ppt

4. **Bagaya M.** Essais de formulation des crèmes et laits dermatologiques à base de beurre de karité raffiné et d'acide Salicylique. [Pharmacy thesis]. University of Ouagadougou; 2014,73 p.

5. **Goulbo O**. Trials of formulations of dermatological creams and ointments based on refined shea butter and betamethasone dipropionate. [Thèse de pharmacie]. Université de Ouagadougou; Ouagadougou 2015,132p.

6. **Toé SL**. Essais de mises au point de formulation de crèmes et laits corporels à base du beurre de karité du Burkina Faso. [Pharmacy thesis]. University of Ouagadougou Ouagadougou 2004, 109p. N^{0} 043.

7. **Lebert O**. Le karité et le henné ; Deux matières premières Africaines à fort pouvoir culturel local utilisées dans les cosmétiques. [Thèse de pharmacie]. University of Nantes; Nantes 2005, 101p. N^{0} 034.

8. **Dale AS.** Burkina Faso: shea butter production reaches 34.2 billion FCFA. Journal le nouvel Afrique 4 August 2020.

9. Mariko ABA. Experimental determination of the required hydrophilic/lipophilic balance of shea butter. [Master thesis]. Université I Pr Joseph Ki- Zerbo, Ouagadougou (Burkina Faso) 2018. 65p. N^{0} 221.

10. Mungo P. Travels in the Interior Districts of Africa: Performed in the Years 1795, 1796, and 1797. With An Account of A Subsequent Mission to That Country in 1805. London (Uk),1806.

11. Zaya P. Les moyens d'améliorer le traitement et le nettoyage du karité, International Development Research Centre. Ottawa (Canada), 1999.

12. Cissé Z. Chemistry of shea kernels and butter. Ouagadougou (Burkina Faso) 1992.

13. Traore AS, Barro A. Changes in the physico-chemical parameters of shea butter as a function of treatment and storage. Burkina Faso, 1991.

14. Institute for the Environment and Agricultural Research. Assessment of 10 years of research: 1988-1998. Programme oléo-protagineux, CNRST, 1998.

15. **Food and Agriculture Organization of the United Nations.** Statistical Data on Shea, UNCTAD Secretariat, 2003

16. **Womeni H.M, Tchagna D.T, Ndjouenkeu R, Kapseu C, Mbiapo F.T, Linder M, Fanni J.J et Parmentier M.** Influence des traitements traditionnels des graines et amandes de karité sur la qualité du beurre. FoodAfrica: Improving Food Systems in sub-Saharan Africa: Responding to a Changing Environment. 2006. 8p

17. **Bernatchez C.** Amélioration de la qualité du produit et des procédés de production du beurre de karité biologique et de la logistique des opérations en Afrique : cas du Burkina Faso. [Thesis]. Québec 2007. 210p.

18. **Ouédraogo 0G.** Medicinal plants and medical practices in Burkina Faso. Cas du Plateau Central. Tome I and II. 320 P. [Thesis in Biochemistry and Microbiology]. FAST, Ouagadougou, 1996; No. 75.

19. **0uédraogo A.** Les produits du karité burkinabé : potentialités, productions, commercialisation, réglementation et procédures d'exportation. PNK, 2000. 128p.

20. **Kpegba K, Kpokanu SA, Simalou O, Novidzro KM and Koumaglo KH.** Evaluation of shea butter production techniques in Togo Int. J. Biol. Chem. Sci. 11(4): 1577-1591, 2017

21. **Sallé G et al.** Le karité une richesse potentielle Bois et forêts des Tropiques.2ème trimestre 1991,228 pp. 11-23.

22. **Nikiema A and Umali BE.** Vitellaria paradoxal CF.Gaertn. PROTA (Plan Resources of tropical Africa). [Online] 2007. C[Citation : 07 June 2011] at http://database.org/PROTAhtml/Vitellaria%20paradoxal_En.html.

23. **Carney J and Elias M.** African Shea Butter: A Feminized Subsidy from Nature, Africa, vol. 77, n° 1, February 2007, pp. 37-62 (ISSN 1750-0184 and 0001-9720, DOI 10.3366/afr.2007.77.1.37, read online [archive], consulted on 3 July 2021

24. **Kuyper HW, Traoré M, Dembelé F and Vellema S.** Analyse d'une plate-forme d'innovation dans la filière karité au Mali, Cahiers Agricultures, vol. 26, n° 4, 1er July 2017, p. 45001 (ISSN 1166-7699 and 1777-5949, DOI 10.1051/cagri/2017029, read online [archive], accessed 3 July 2021)

25. **Fold N, Reenberg A.** In the shadow of the 'chocolate war': local marketing of shea nut products around Tenkodogo, Burkina Faso". Geografisk Tidsskrift / Danish Journal of Geography Special Issue 1999. 2: 113-123.

26. **Elias M, Saussey M.** 'The Gift that keeps on giving': unveiling the paradoxes of fairness trade shea butter". Sociologia Ruralis 2013, 53(2): 158-179.

27. **Masters ET, Yidana JA and Lovett PN. Error ! Invalid hyperlink reference.** [archive], Vol. 55 2004/4, at www.fao.org, International Journal of Forestry and Forest Industries, 2004; No. 219 (accessed 7 July 2021) ;

28. **Rousseau K.** Political ecology du karité - Relations de pouvoir et changements sociaux et environnementaux liés à la mondialisation du commerce des amandes de karité - Cas de l'Ouest du Burkina Faso [PhD thesis], AgroParis Tech, June 2016

29. **Davrieux F, Allal F, Piombo G, Kelly B, Okulo JB, Thiam M, Diallo OB, Bouvet J-M.** Near Infrared Spectroscopy for High-Throughput Characterization of Shea Tree (Vitellaria paradoxa) Nut Fat Profiles [archive]. Journal of Agricultural and Food Chemistry 2010. 58:7811-7819.

30. **Maranz S, Wiesman Z, Bisgaard J, Bianchi G.** Germplasm resources of Vitellaria paradoxa based on variations in fat composition across the species distribution range", Agroforestry Systems, vol. 60, n° 1, 1er January 2004, pp. 71-76 (ISSN 1572-9680, DOI 10.1023/B:AGFO.00000094 06.19593.90, online reading [archive], accessed 14 July 2021).

31. **Alander J.** Shea butter-a multifunctional ingredient for food and cosmetics. Lipid Technol 2004. 16. 202-205.

32. **Lin T-K, Zhong L and Santiago JL.** 'Anti-Inflammatory and Skin Barrier Repair Effects of Topical Application of Some Plant Oils', International Journal of Molecular Sciences, vol. 19, n° 1, 27 December 2017 (ISSN 1422-0067, PMID 29280987, PMCID 5796020,
DOI 10.3390/ijms19010070, read online [archive], accessed 12 July 2021)

33. **Maranz S and Wissman Z.** The Phyto-Oleochemical Laboratory, The Institutes for Applied Research, Ben-Gurion University of the Negev, Israel), "Influence of Climate on the Tocopherol Content of Shea Butter", Journal of Agricultural and Food Chemistry 2004. 52(10):2934-2937 (ISSN 0021-8561 and 1520-5118, DOI 10.1021/jf035194r.

34. **Akihisa T, Kojima N, Katoh N and Uchimura Y.** Triterpene alcohol and fatty acid composition of shea nuts from seven African countries ", Journal of Oleo Science, vol. 59, n° 7, 2010, p. 351-360 (ISSN 1347-3352, PMID 20513968.

35. **Di Vincenzo D, Maranz S, Serraiocco A and Vito R.** Regional variation in shea butter lipid and triterpene composition in four African countries", Journal of Agricultural and Food Chemistry, vol. 53, n° 19, 21 September 2005, pp. 7473-7479 (ISSN 0021-8561, PMID 16159175, DOI 10.1021/jf0509759, read online [archive], accessed 13 July 2021).

36. **Davrieux F, Allal F, Piombo G and Kelly B.** Near infrared spectroscopy for high-throughput characterization of Shea tree (Vitellaria paradoxa) nut fat profiles", Journal of Agricultural and Food Chemistry, vol. 58, n° 13, 14 July 2010, pp. 7811-7819 (ISSN 1520-5118, PMID 20518501, DOI 10.1021/jf100409v, online reading [archive], accessed 13 July 2021).

37. **Digital Institute.** Chapter 10: Mali in the shea industry. [Site int] available at https://www.institut-numerique.org/chapitre-10-le-mali-dans-la-filiere-karite- 51c2d0 f1b4296 consulted on 06.07.21 at 01h20.

38. **Joutel B**. Commodity chain analysis, a development tool for NGOs in the South. The

case of Malian shea. [Dissertation] Université Pierre Mendès France 2011. Available at https://www.memoireonline.com/08/13/7309/L-analyse-de-filiere-un-outil-de- developpement-pour-les-ONG-dans-le-sud.html

39. **Nacoulma OG.** Communication on shea butter, Ouagadougou, 2000.

40. **Dupont J.** Microfluidic emulsification processes: Potential for pharmaceuticals. [Pharmacy thesis]. University of Lille 2; 2017. 118p.

41. **Brochette P.** Emulsification - Elaboration and study of emulsions, Techniques de l'ingénieur, ref: J2150 V2, 2013.

42. **Deepak S, Sanjay K, Piyush A**. Recent advancement, technology & applications of the multiple emulsions, Innovare Journal of Health sciences 2013, 1(1).

43. **Marcel B, Meinders J, Van Vliet T.** The role of interfacial rheological properties on Ostwald ripening in emulsions, Advances in Colloid and Interface Science. 2004, 108-109,;119-26

44. **Koroleva M, Tokarev A, Yurtov E**. (). Simulation of flocculation in W/O emulsions and experimental study, Colloids and Surfaces, Physicochemical and Engineering Aspects 2015, 481:237-243.

45. **Poux M and Cancelier JP.** Emulsification processes - Techniques and equipment, Techniques de l'ingénieur 2004, ref J2153 V1

46. **Garti N, Bisperink C.** Double emulsions: progress and applications, Curr. Opin. Colloid Interface Science. 1998. Vol. 3: 657-667p

47. **Klahn JK, Janssen JJM, Vaessen GEJ, De Swart R, Agterof WGM.** On the escape process during phase inversion of an emulsion, Colloid Surf. A: Physicochem. Eng. Aspects. 2002; vol. 210: 167-181p

48. **Van der Graaf S., Schröen C.G.P.H., Boom R.M.** Preparation of double emulsions by membrane emulsification-a review, Journal of Membrane Science. 2005; 251:7-15

49. **Charpentier J.C.** Intensification des procédés, Techniques de l'ingénieur. 2016, ref J7000 V1

50. **Raymond C Rowe. Paul J Sheskey. Sia^n C Owen.** Handbook of Pharmaceutical Excipients. Fifth edition. London, UK. 2005. 945p

51. **A.Le Hir. J.-C. Chaumiel et Al.** Pharmacie Galénique Bonnes pratiques de fabrication des médicaments. 10° edition, 2016. 173p

52. **M.-L. Dupasquier, A. Nazari et AL,** CDIEC. Cosmetic formulation, emulsions, Université of Nice Sophia Antipolis. Available at https://ressources.unisciel.fr/formulation_cosmetique/co/1-1.html

APPENDICES

Name: *Fonga Noutchia*

First name: *Placide Nelson*

Material Safety Data Sheet

Title of thesis: *Emulsifying properties of shea butter produced in Mali*

City of defence: *Bamako*

Country of origin: *Cameroon*

Depository: *Library of the Faculty of Medicine, Pharmacy and Odontostomatology (FMOS, FAPH) in Bamako*

Sector of interest: *Galenics and Cosmetics.*

Summary:

Introduction: *Shea butter, known for thousands of years, is a highly prized resource among African populations, who already used it as a plant medicine for its anti-inflammatory, anti-haemorrhoidal, relaxing, cough-relieving, antioxidant and healing properties. It was also used as a food and raw material in the manufacture of soaps for domestic use.*

Objective: *To study the emulsifying properties of shea butter produced in Mali.*

Methodology: *We carried out an experimental and descriptive study of Malian shea butter from the Bougouni region. We used a one-dimensional scanning method of shea butter to determine the appropriate proportions needed for the butter to form stable emulsions with water without the addition of any stabilising agent. The quantities of water ranged from 0 to 90% in the formulae with scales of 10 to 10.*

Results: *At the end of the preparation, the creams one (01) to four (04) and eight (08) were stable and fluid 2h after emulsification. Creams five (05) to seven (07) were stable and thick. All the creams had a milky white appearance and were semi-solid to solid in consistency. We therefore deduce that the globule sizes were between one (01) and five (05) µm, which corresponds to an average emulsion. All our emulsions were not washable with water and were of the W/O type.The appearance of the creams evolved differently over the course of the temples. The most stable after 90 days were creams one (01) to seven (07). The proportions of creams one (01) to seven (07) ranged from 0 to 60% water.Shea butter can therefore incorporate up to 60% water without showing signs of instability. after 90J as described above.****Conclusion*** : *Composed largely of oleic and stearic acids, shea butter combined with water produces stable emulsions in well-defined proportions. This characteristic gives it emulsifying properties, so it can absorb almost twice its weight in water.*

Key words : **Emulsifying properties, shea butter, Mali,**

GALEN'S OATH

 I swear, in the presence of the masters of the faculty, the councillors of the Ordre des pharmacists and my colleagues:
 To honour those who have instructed me in the precepts of my art, and to thank them for their support. to show my gratitude by remaining faithful to their teaching;
 To practise my profession conscientiously in the interests of public health and to comply not only with the legislation in force, but also with the rules of honour, probity and selflessness.
 Never to forget my responsibility and duties towards patients and their human dignity.

 Under no circumstances will I agree to use my knowledge and condition to corrupt morals and encourage criminal acts.
 May men esteem me if I am faithful to my promises.
 May I be shamed and despised by my colleagues if I fail to do so.

I swear!

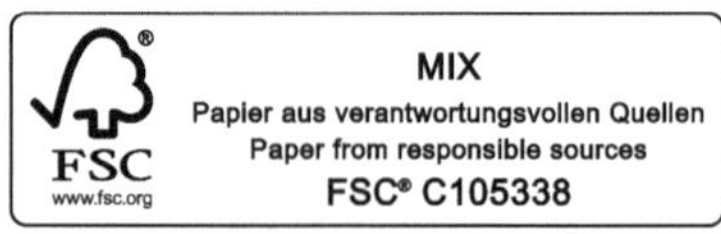

Printed by Books on Demand GmbH, Norderstedt / Germany